# NO GALLBLADDER GUIDE AND COOK BOOK FOR BEGINNERS

## A Comprehensive Recovery Plan To Managing Your Health and Meals After Gallbladder Removal

BY

## EDITH BERNHARDT

# TABLE OF CONTENTS


INTRODUCTION..................................................... 5

CHAPTER ONE: PREPARING FOR THE POST-SURGERY JOURNEY................................. 7

Different Surgical Techniques and Their Implications:............................................... 8

Expected Recovery Timeline and Postoperative Care:.................................................. 10

Preparing Your Home Environment................11

Navigating Postoperative Pain and Discomfort... 15


After gallbladder removal surgery, experiencing some degree of pain and discomfort is normal as your body heals from the surgical procedure. Understanding how to manage postoperative pain and discomfort effectively is essential for promoting recovery and ensuring a smoother transition back to daily activities. This section provides insights into pain management strategies, recognizing normal versus concerning symptoms, and tips for optimising comfort during the initial recovery period........ 15


Establishing Open Communication with Healthcare Providers.....................................19

Emotional Preparation and Support Systems. 23

Planning for Dietary Changes........................ 27

CHAPTER TWO: NUTRITIONAL GUIDELINES AND DIETARY CONSIDERATIONS.................... 31

Understanding Dietary Modifications.............. 31

Managing Food Intolerances and Sensitivities After Gallbladder Removal.............................40

**CHAPTER THREE: TIPS FOR DIGESTIVE HEALTH AND COMFORT**.................................47

Mindful Eating Practices....................47

Balancing Macronutrients.....................50

Achieving a balance of macronutrients—proteins, carbohydrates, and fats—in your diet is essential for supporting overall health, promoting satiety, and optimizing digestion after gallbladder removal surgery. Here's how you can effectively balance macronutrients in your meals:........................50

Managing Fibre Intake.................... 53

Hydration Strategies....................56

Incorporating Digestive Aids.................... 59

Regular Physical Activity....................62

Establishing a Consistent Sleep Routine:....... 66

Gradual Introduction of Trigger Foods........... 68

**CHAPTER FOUR: DELICIOUS RECIPES FOR GALLBLADDER-FRIENDLY MEALS**.................. 71

Breakfast Delights.................... 71

Lunchtime Favourites....................79

Dinner Creations.................... 84

Snacks and Sides.................... 87

**CHAPTER FIVE: COPING WITH CHALLENGES AND COMMON CONCERNS**....................93

Managing Digestive Discomfort.................... 93

Coping with Emotional and Psychological Effects After Gallbladder Removal Surgery.. 100

Adapting to Lifestyle Changes After Gallbladder Removal Surgery.................... 103

Fostering Resilience and Optimism After Gallbladder Removal Surgery.................... 107

**CONCLUSION: EMBRACING A VIBRANT LIFESTYLE WITHOUT A GALLBLADDER....... 111**

# INTRODUCTION

The decision to undergo gallbladder removal surgery marks a significant milestone in one's health journey. Whether prompted by gallstones, gallbladder inflammation, or other related conditions, this surgical procedure often brings relief from debilitating symptoms. However, it also initiates a new phase in your relationship with food and well-being.

In this introductory chapter, we embark on a journey to understand the nuances of life after gallbladder removal. We delve into the functions of the gallbladder, its role in digestion, and the implications of its absence. Moreover, we explore the common reasons for gallbladder removal, empowering you with knowledge to navigate this transition with confidence.

As we embark on this exploration, it's essential to acknowledge the physical and emotional adjustments that accompany surgical intervention. From adapting to dietary changes to managing potential digestive challenges, each aspect of post-surgery life requires attention and understanding.

Throughout this guide and cookbook, we aim to provide comprehensive support, equipping you with practical insights, nutritional guidance, and flavorful recipes tailored to your unique needs. By fostering a deeper understanding of life after gallbladder removal, we strive to empower you to embrace wellness and vitality in your daily life. Let's embark on this transformative journey together.

# CHAPTER ONE: PREPARING FOR THE POST-SURGERY JOURNEY

Preparing for  post-surgery phase after gallbladder removal requires thoughtful preparation and a proactive approach to ensure a smooth and successful recovery. This chapter serves as your guide, offering valuable insights into the practical aspects of preparing for the journey ahead.

Gallbladder removal surgery, medically termed ***cholecystectomy***, is a procedure aimed at relieving symptoms caused by gallstones, gallbladder inflammation (cholecystitis), or other gallbladder-related issues. This surgical intervention entails careful planning and execution, involving various steps and considerations for both patients and healthcare professionals.

## Overview of Gallbladder Removal Surgery:

Gallbladder removal surgery is typically recommended when gallstones cause persistent pain, inflammation, or complications such as infections or blockages in the bile ducts. The gallbladder is a small organ located beneath the liver, responsible for storing and concentrating bile produced by the liver. Bile aids in the digestion of fats in the small intestine. During cholecystectomy, the surgeon removes the gallbladder through one of several surgical techniques, depending on factors such as the patient's medical history, the severity of the condition, and the surgeon's expertise.

## Different Surgical Techniques and Their Implications:

**1. Laparoscopic Cholecystectomy:** Laparoscopic cholecystectomy is the preferred approach for most cases of gallbladder removal.In this minimally invasive procedure, the surgeon makes several small incisions in the abdomen and inserts a laparoscope (a thin tube with a camera) and specialised surgical instruments.

The laparoscope provides a magnified view of the internal organs on a monitor, allowing the surgeon to carefully dissect and remove the gallbladder with minimal trauma to surrounding tissues.Laparoscopic cholecystectomy is associated with shorter hospital stays, reduced postoperative pain, and faster recovery times compared to open surgery.

## 2. Open Cholecystectomy:

Open cholecystectomy involves making a larger incision in the abdomen to access the gallbladder directly.

This approach may be necessary in cases where laparoscopic surgery is not feasible, such as in the presence of severe inflammation, scarring from previous surgeries, or anatomical variations. Although open cholecystectomy may result in a longer recovery period and increased postoperative discomfort, it remains a viable option in certain circumstances.

# Expected Recovery Timeline and Postoperative Care:

Following gallbladder removal surgery, patients typically experience a period of recovery and adjustment as their bodies adapt to the absence of the gallbladder. The recovery timeline may vary depending on factors such as the surgical technique used, individual health status, and adherence to postoperative guidelines.

**Common aspects of postoperative care and recovery include:**

**1. *Pain management*:**
Patients may experience discomfort or pain at the incision sites, which can be managed with medications prescribed by the healthcare provider.

**2.*Dietary modifications:*** In the initial postoperative period, patients may be advised to follow a temporary low-fat diet to minimise digestive disturbances and aid in healing.

**3.*Physical activity:*** While rest is important during the immediate postoperative period, patients are encouraged to gradually resume light activities and mobility as tolerated.

**4.Follow-up appointments:** Regular follow-up visits with the healthcare provider allow for monitoring of recovery progress, assessment of surgical incisions, and addressing any concerns or complications that may arise.

## Preparing Your Home Environment

Creating a conducive and supportive environment for recovery is paramount following gallbladder removal surgery. Your home environment plays a crucial role in facilitating a smooth and comfortable recovery process. This section outlines practical steps and considerations for preparing your home environment to optimise your post-surgery experience.

**Creating a Comfortable and Supportive Space for Recovery includes:**

**1. Restful Sleeping Area:** Ensure your bedroom provides a comfortable and restful environment conducive to quality sleep. Consider investing in supportive pillows and bedding to promote proper alignment and minimize discomfort.

**2. *Relaxation Zones:*** Designate areas within your home where you can engage in relaxation and leisure activities, such as reading, listening to music, or practising mindfulness techniques.

**3. *Clear Pathways:*** Remove clutter and obstacles from hallways and walkways to prevent tripping hazards and facilitate safe movement throughout your home.

**4. *Temperature Control:*** Maintain a comfortable temperature within your home to promote relaxation and alleviate discomfort during the recovery period.

**Practical Considerations for Post-Surgery Living Arrangements:**

**1. *Accessibility:*** Arrange commonly used items and essentials within easy reach to minimise the need for bending, stretching, or reaching overhead.

**2. *Bathroom Accessibility:*** Ensure that your bathroom is easily accessible and equipped with supportive handrails or grab bars to assist with mobility and stability.

**3. *Assistance:*** If possible, arrange for assistance from family members, friends, or caregivers during the initial stages of recovery to help with daily tasks and provide emotional support.

**4. *Transportation:*** Plan for transportation to and from medical appointments, pharmacy visits, and other essential errands, especially if driving is restricted during the recovery period.

**Necessary Supplies and Aids for Easing Daily Activities:**

**1.*Medication:*** Ensure that you have a sufficient supply of prescribed medications, pain relievers, and any other postoperative medications recommended by your healthcare provider.

**2. *Wound Care Supplies:*** Stock up on wound care supplies, including sterile gauze, adhesive bandages, and antiseptic solutions, to maintain proper hygiene and facilitate healing of surgical incisions.

**3. *Mobility Aids:*** Consider using assistive devices such as walkers, canes, or shower chairs to enhance mobility and safety, particularly if you experience weakness or instability during the recovery process.

**4. *Nutritional Support:*** Stock your kitchen with nutritious foods and beverages that align with your postoperative dietary guidelines, including easily digestible options such as soups, broths, and soft fruits.

By proactively addressing these considerations and making necessary preparations, you can create a supportive and nurturing environment that promotes healing and enhances your overall well-being during the post-surgery recovery period. Remember to communicate openly with your healthcare team and enlist the support of loved ones to ensure a smooth transition and successful recovery journey.

# Navigating Postoperative Pain and Discomfort

After gallbladder removal surgery, experiencing some degree of pain and discomfort is normal as your body heals from the surgical procedure. Understanding how to manage postoperative pain and discomfort effectively is essential for promoting recovery and ensuring a smoother transition back to daily activities. This section provides insights into pain management strategies, recognizing normal versus concerning symptoms, and tips for optimising comfort during the initial recovery period.

**Pain Management Strategies and Medications:**
*1. Follow Prescribed Pain Medications:* Your healthcare provider will prescribe pain medications to help alleviate discomfort during the recovery process. It's mandatory l to take these

medications as directed to manage pain effectively.

**2. *Use Ice Packs:*** Applying ice packs to the surgical site can help reduce inflammation and numb the area, providing temporary relief from pain and swelling.

**3. *Practice Relaxation Techniques:*** Engage in relaxation techniques such as deep breathing, meditation, or guided imagery to help distract your mind from pain and promote a sense of calm.

**4. *Positioning:*** Experiment with different body positions, such as lying down, sitting, or reclining, to find the most comfortable posture that alleviates pressure on the surgical incisions.

**5. *Gentle Movement:*** Engage in light stretching and gentle movement exercises as tolerated to prevent stiffness and promote circulation. However, avoid strenuous activities that may exacerbate pain or discomfort.

**Recognizing Normal Versus Concerning Symptoms:**

**1. *Expected Pain Levels:*** It's normal to experience varying levels of pain and discomfort in the days following surgery. However, if your pain becomes severe or persists despite taking prescribed pain medications, contact your healthcare provider promptly.

**2. *Surgical Incisions:*** Monitor the appearance of your surgical incisions for signs of infection, such as redness, swelling, warmth, or drainage. Contact your healthcare provider if you notice any concerning changes in the incision sites.

**3. *Fever:*** A low-grade fever is common in the immediate postoperative period. However, if you develop a fever above 100.4°F (38°C) or experience chills, this could indicate an infection and should be reported to your healthcare provider.

**Tips for Optimising Comfort During the Initial Recovery Period:**

**1. *Rest and Sleep:*** Prioritise rest and ensure adequate sleep to promote healing and rejuvenation. Use supportive pillows or cushions to maintain a comfortable sleeping position.

**2. *Hydration:*** Stay hydrated by drinking plenty of fluids, such as water, herbal teas, or electrolyte solutions, to prevent dehydration and promote overall well-being.

**3. *Dietary Modifications:*** Follow your healthcare provider's dietary recommendations, including consuming light, easily digestible foods to minimise gastrointestinal discomfort.

**4. *Supportive Garments:*** Consider wearing loose-fitting, comfortable clothing that does not constrict or irritate the surgical incisions.

**5. *Emotional Support:*** Seek emotional support from friends, family members, or support groups to cope with any emotional challenges or concerns during the recovery process.

By implementing these strategies and remaining vigilant in monitoring your symptoms, you can navigate postoperative pain and discomfort more effectively while promoting a smoother recovery journey. Remember to communicate openly with your healthcare provider about your pain levels and any concerns you may have to ensure appropriate management and support.

# Establishing Open Communication with Healthcare Providers

Building a strong and open line of communication with your healthcare providers is crucial for ensuring optimal care and support throughout the postoperative recovery period following gallbladder removal surgery. Effective communication allows you to address concerns, seek clarification on post-surgery expectations, and stay informed about your progress. This section highlights key strategies for fostering communication with your medical team.

### Building a Rapport with Your Medical Team:

*1. Active Listening:* Actively listen to your healthcare providers during preoperative consultations, postoperative appointments, and follow-up visits. Take notes and ask questions to ensure that you understand the information provided.

**2. *Express Your Concerns:*** Share any concerns, anxieties, or questions you may have with your medical team in a clear and respectful manner. Your healthcare providers are there to support you and address your needs.

**3. *Advocate for Yourself:*** Be an active participant in your healthcare journey by advocating for your well-being and expressing your preferences regarding treatment options, pain management strategies, and postoperative care.

**4. *Establish Trust:*** Foster a trusting relationship with your healthcare providers by being honest and transparent about your symptoms, experiences, and recovery progress. Trust forms the foundation of effective communication and collaborative decision-making.

**Addressing Concerns and Seeking Clarification on Post-Surgery Expectations:**

**1. *Ask Questions:*** Don't hesitate to ask questions about your post-surgery care plan, including dietary restrictions, activity limitations, and potential complications to watch for. Seek clarification on any information that is unclear or confusing.

**2. *Discuss Pain Management:*** Talk to your healthcare provider about your pain levels and preferences for pain management. Work together to develop a pain management plan that addresses your needs while minimising potential side effects.

**3. *Inquire About Recovery Milestones:*** Discuss realistic expectations for the recovery process, including anticipated milestones, timeline for resuming normal activities, and signs of progress.

**4. *Explore Resources:*** Inquire about educational resources, support groups, or online forums where you can find additional information and connect with others who have undergone similar experiences.

**Scheduling Follow-Up Appointments and Monitoring Progress:**

**1. Follow-Up Visits:** Schedule follow-up appointments with your healthcare provider as recommended to monitor your progress, assess surgical incisions, and address any concerns or complications that may arise.

**2. Keep Track of Symptoms:** Keep a journal or diary to track your symptoms, medication use, dietary intake, and any notable changes in your condition. This information can help you communicate effectively with your healthcare provider during follow-up visits.

**3. Report Changes Promptly:** If you experience new or worsening symptoms, such as persistent pain, fever, nausea, vomiting, or changes in bowel habits, contact your healthcare provider promptly to discuss your concerns and determine the appropriate course of action.

By establishing open communication with your healthcare providers, you can navigate the postoperative recovery process with confidence, receive personalised care and support, and achieve optimal outcomes following gallbladder removal surgery.

Remember that your medical team is there to guide you every step of the way, so don't hesitate to reach out for assistance whenever needed.

## Emotional Preparation and Support Systems

Preparing for gallbladder removal surgery involves more than just physical readiness—it also requires emotional preparedness and the establishment of robust support systems to navigate the challenges and transitions that accompany surgical intervention. This section delves deeper into recognizing and addressing the emotional aspects of surgery, building a support network of friends and family, and exploring resources for mental and emotional well-being.

**Recognizing and Addressing Emotional Aspects of Surgery:**
*1. Acknowledge Feelings:* It's normal to experience a range of emotions before undergoing surgery, including anxiety, fear, uncertainty, and even relief. Acknowledge

and validate your feelings without judgement, recognizing that they are a natural response to significant life events.

**2. *Educate Yourself:*** Educate yourself about the surgical procedure, recovery process, and potential outcomes to alleviate fears and uncertainties. Ask your healthcare provider for information, read reputable sources, and seek guidance from support groups or online forums.

**3. *Practice Self-Compassion:*** Be kind to yourself and practice self-compassion as you navigate the emotional challenges of surgery. Allow yourself to feel and process your emotions without self-criticism or judgement.

**4. *Seek Professional Support:*** If you find yourself struggling to cope with overwhelming emotions or anxiety related to surgery, consider seeking support from a mental health professional, such as a therapist or counsellor. Therapy can provide a safe space to express how you feel, and develop coping strategies, and gain perspective on your experiences.

**Building a Support Network of Friends and Family:**

*1. Open Communication:* Communicate openly with your friends and family members about your upcoming surgery, including your feelings, concerns, and needs. Share information about the procedure and how they can best support you during the recovery process.

*2. Practical Assistance:* Enlist the help of friends and family members in coordinating transportation to and from the hospital, running errands, preparing meals, and providing assistance with household chores during the initial stages of recovery.

*3. Emotional Support:* Lean on your support network for emotional support and encouragement throughout the surgical journey. Express gratitude for their presence and reassure them of your appreciation for their support.

*4. Set Boundaries:* Be clear about your boundaries and preferences regarding visitors, phone calls, and communication during the recovery period. Prioritise your needs and well-being as you navigate the postoperative transition.

**Exploring Resources for Mental and Emotional Well-Being:**

***1. Support Groups:*** Consider joining support groups or online communities for individuals who have undergone gallbladder removal surgery or other medical procedures. These groups can provide valuable insights, camaraderie, and emotional support from individuals who understand your experiences firsthand.

***2. Mindfulness Practices:*** Explore mindfulness techniques such as meditation, deep breathing exercises, guided imagery, or progressive muscle relaxation to promote relaxation, reduce stress, and enhance emotional well-being.

***3. Holistic Therapies:*** Explore holistic therapies such as acupuncture, massage therapy, yoga, or aromatherapy to support your overall well-being and promote relaxation during the recovery process.

***4. Self-Care Activities:*** Prioritise self-care activities that nourish your mind, body, and spirit, such as spending time in nature, engaging in creative pursuits, practising gratitude, or indulging in hobbies that bring you joy and fulfilment.

# Planning for Dietary Changes

Adjusting to dietary changes following gallbladder removal surgery is a crucial aspect of the postoperative recovery process. This section provides an introduction to post-gallbladder removal dietary adjustments, guidance on easing into a modified eating plan, and insights into understanding potential food intolerances and sensitivities.

**Introduction to Post-Gallbladder Removal Dietary Adjustments:**
*1. Importance of Dietary Changes:* After gallbladder removal surgery, your body's ability to store and release bile, which aids in the digestion of fats, may be compromised. As a result, adjustments to your diet are necessary to prevent digestive discomfort and promote optimal nutrient absorption.
*2. Dietary Guidelines:* Your healthcare provider may recommend dietary

modifications to accommodate the absence
of the gallbladder and minimise the risk of
digestive symptoms such as bloating, gas,
diarrhoea, or indigestion. These guidelines
may include reducing intake of high-fat
foods, increasing consumption of fibre-rich
foods, and eating smaller, more frequent
meals throughout the day.

**Guidance on Easing into a Modified Eating Plan:**
*1. Gradual Transition:* Ease into a
modified eating plan gradually, allowing
your body time to adjust to dietary changes.
Start by incorporating easily digestible
foods such as lean proteins, whole grains,
fruits, and vegetables into your meals.
*2. Emphasise Low-Fat Options:*
Choose lean sources of protein such as
poultry, fish, tofu, and legumes, and opt for
low-fat dairy products to minimise the
strain on your digestive system.
*3. Monitor Portion Sizes*: Pay attention
to portion sizes and avoid overeating, as
large meals can overwhelm your digestive
system and lead to discomfort. Aim for
smaller, more frequent meals and snacks to

support optimal digestion and nutrient absorption.

**4. Stay Hydrated:** Drink plenty of fluids throughout the day, including water, herbal teas, and clear broths, to stay hydrated and support digestive health.

**Understanding Potential Food Intolerances and Sensitivities:**

**1. Keep a Food Diary:** Keep track of your dietary intake and any associated symptoms in a food diary to identify potential triggers for digestive discomfort. Note any foods that seem to exacerbate symptoms or cause gastrointestinal distress.

**2. Common Trigger Foods:** Certain foods may be more likely to trigger digestive symptoms in individuals who have undergone gallbladder removal surgery. These may include high-fat foods, spicy foods, fried foods, dairy products, caffeine, and carbonated beverages.

**3. Experiment with Elimination:** Experiment with eliminating potential trigger foods from your diet to determine whether they contribute to digestive symptoms. Gradually reintroduce these foods one at a time to assess your tolerance and identify any specific triggers.

**4. Consult with a Dietitian:** Consider consulting with a registered dietitian or nutritionist who can provide personalised dietary guidance tailored to your individual needs, preferences, and digestive tolerance levels.

By proactively planning for dietary changes, easing into a modified eating plan, and understanding potential food intolerances and sensitivities, you can support digestive health, minimise discomfort, and optimise your overall well-being following gallbladder removal surgery. Remember to listen to your body's cues, prioritise nutrient-rich foods, and seek professional guidance as needed to navigate the postoperative dietary transition effectively.

By proactively addressing these key aspects, you'll lay the foundation for a smoother transition into the post-surgery phase.

# CHAPTER TWO: NUTRITIONAL GUIDELINES AND DIETARY CONSIDERATIONS

Navigating the post-gallbladder removal dietary landscape requires a thoughtful approach to ensure optimal digestion, nutrient absorption, and overall well-being. In this chapter, we explore essential nutritional guidelines and dietary considerations tailored to support your health and comfort following gallbladder removal surgery. From understanding dietary modifications to incorporating nutrient-rich foods into your meals, we aim to empower you with the knowledge and tools needed to make informed choices and thrive in your postoperative journey.

## Understanding Dietary Modifications

Dietary modifications play a crucial role in promoting digestive health and overall

well-being after gallbladder removal
surgery. Here's a deeper look at the dietary
adjustments necessary for thriving without
a gallbladder:

**Overview of Dietary Adjustments:**
Following gallbladder removal surgery, the
body's ability to store and release bile, a
digestive fluid produced by the liver, is
altered. Without a gallbladder, bile is
continuously released into the digestive
system, which can impact the way fats are
digested. As a result, dietary adjustments
are essential to minimise digestive
discomfort and support optimal digestion.

**Importance of Reducing Intake of
High-Fat Foods:**
High-fat foods can be challenging to digest
without the presence of a gallbladder.
Consuming large amounts of fat can lead to
symptoms such as bloating, gas, and
diarrhoea. Therefore, it's important to
reduce the intake of high-fat foods,
including fried foods, fatty cuts of meat,
processed snacks, and rich desserts.
Instead, focus on incorporating healthy fats

from sources such as avocados, nuts, seeds, and olive oil in moderate amounts.

**Emphasising Fiber-Rich Foods:**
Fiber plays a crucial role in promoting digestive health and regularity, which is especially important after gallbladder removal surgery. Fibre helps to regulate bowel movements, prevent constipation, and support overall digestive function. Incorporate fibre-rich foods such as fruits, vegetables, whole grains, legumes, and nuts into your meals and snacks. However, it's important to gradually increase fibre intake to allow your digestive system to adjust.

**Incorporating Lean Proteins, Complex Carbohydrates, and Healthy Fats:**
A well-balanced diet is key to supporting overall health and nutrition after gallbladder surgery. Aim to include lean proteins such as poultry, fish, tofu, and legumes in your meals to provide essential amino acids for muscle repair and maintenance. Incorporate complex carbohydrates from sources such as whole

grains, vegetables, and fruits to provide sustained energy levels and promote satiety. Additionally, include healthy fats from sources like avocados, olive oil, nuts, and seeds to support heart health and enhance the absorption of fat-soluble vitamins.

By understanding the importance of dietary modifications and making mindful food choices, you can optimise digestion, minimise discomfort, and support your overall health and well-being after gallbladder removal surgery. Listen to your body's cues, experiment with different foods, and consult with healthcare professionals or registered dietitians for personalised guidance and support on your dietary journey.

## Adopting a Modified Eating Plan

Embarking on a modified eating plan after gallbladder removal is a gradual process that allows your body to adjust to the changes in digestive function. Here's a closer look at the key considerations for successfully adopting a modified eating plan:

### Guidance on Easing Into a Modified Eating Plan Gradually:
Transitioning to a modified eating plan is most effective when done gradually. Start by introducing changes to your diet slowly, allowing your digestive system to adapt. Begin with small adjustments, such as incorporating more fiber-rich foods, lean proteins, and healthy fats. This gradual approach enables you to monitor how your body responds to specific dietary modifications.

### Emphasising Portion Control and Eating Smaller, More Frequent Meals:
Portion control becomes paramount after gallbladder removal. Instead of consuming large meals, opt for smaller, more frequent meals throughout the day. This approach minimises the demand on your digestive system, preventing overwhelming surges of bile and reducing the likelihood of digestive discomfort. Aim for balanced meals that

include lean proteins, complex carbohydrates, and healthy fats to provide sustained energy.

## Strategies for Choosing Low-Fat Options:

Since the gallbladder is responsible for storing and releasing bile to aid in fat digestion, choosing low-fat options is crucial. Opt for lean cuts of meat, trim visible fats from poultry, and select low-fat dairy products. Experiment with cooking methods such as baking, grilling, or steaming instead of frying. Incorporating sources of healthy fats, such as avocados, nuts, and olive oil, in moderate amounts can provide essential nutrients without overwhelming the digestive system.

## Minimising Dietary Triggers for Digestive Symptoms:

Identify and minimise dietary triggers that may exacerbate digestive symptoms. Common triggers include spicy foods, greasy or fried dishes, and certain dairy products. Pay attention to how your body reacts to different foods, keeping a food diary if necessary. Individual tolerance levels vary, so it's essential to tailor your diet to your specific needs, avoiding foods that may cause discomfort or digestive distress.

**Tips for Staying Hydrated and Maintaining Adequate Fluid Intake:** Adequate hydration is essential for supporting digestion, preventing constipation, and ensuring overall well-being. Drink plenty of water throughout the day, at least eight glasses. Opt for hydrating foods like water-rich fruits and vegetables. However, be mindful of your beverage choices, as some individuals may find that caffeinated and carbonated drinks can contribute to discomfort. Adjust your fluid intake based on your individual needs and listen to your body's signals for thirst.

## Prioritising Nutrient-Rich Foods for Optimal Health After Gallbladder Removal

Incorporating nutrient-rich foods into your diet is essential for supporting overall health, promoting digestion, and enhancing well-being after gallbladder removal surgery. Here's a closer look at how you can prioritize nutrient-rich foods to optimize your postoperative nutrition:

**Identifying Nutrient-Rich Foods:**
Nutrient-rich foods are packed with essential vitamins, minerals, antioxidants, and dietary fibre that are vital for supporting various bodily functions. These foods provide the building blocks necessary for tissue repair, immune function, energy production, and overall vitality. By focusing on nutrient-dense options, you can fuel your body with the essential nutrients it needs to thrive.

**Incorporating Fruits and Vegetables:**
Fruits and vegetables are rich sources of vitamins, minerals, and dietary fibre, making them essential components of a balanced diet. Aim to include a colourful variety of fruits and vegetables in your meals and snacks to maximise nutrient

intake. Leafy greens, berries, citrus fruits, cruciferous vegetables, and root vegetables are excellent choices that provide a wide array of health-promoting nutrients.

## Choosing Whole Grains and Legumes:

Whole grains and legumes are valuable sources of complex carbohydrates, protein, fibre, and essential nutrients. Incorporate whole grains such as quinoa, brown rice, oats, barley, and whole wheat into your meals to provide sustained energy and promote satiety. Legumes, including beans, lentils, chickpeas, and peas, are excellent plant-based protein sources that contribute to overall health and digestive function.

## Selecting Lean Sources of Protein:

Protein is essential for muscle repair, immune function, and satiety. Choose lean sources of protein such as poultry, fish, tofu, tempeh, beans, and legumes to support muscle health and promote feelings of fullness. Incorporating a variety of protein sources into your diet ensures that you receive a complete array of amino acids necessary for optimal health and well-being.

**Exploring Healthy Fats:**
Healthy fats play a crucial role in supporting cell structure, hormone production, brain function, and nutrient absorption. Incorporate sources of healthy fats such as avocados, nuts, seeds, and olive oil into your meals to provide essential fatty acids and enhance flavor. These heart-healthy fats not only contribute to overall well-being but also help to promote satiety and satisfaction with meals.

# Managing Food Intolerances and Sensitivities After Gallbladder Removal

Food intolerances and sensitivities can complicate the postoperative journey after gallbladder removal surgery, leading to digestive discomfort and other symptoms. Here are some strategies to help identify and manage food intolerances and sensitivities effectively:

## Strategies for Identifying Potential Food Intolerances and Sensitivities:

**1.** Pay close attention to how your body reacts to different foods and ingredients after gallbladder removal surgery.

**2.** Be mindful of symptoms such as bloating, gas, abdominal pain, diarrhoea, or nausea that may indicate a food intolerance or sensitivity.

**3.** Keep track of your dietary intake and associated symptoms using a food diary or journal.

## Keeping a Food Diary:

**1.** Maintain a detailed record of everything you eat and drink, as well as any symptoms experienced afterward.

**2.** Note the time of day, portion sizes, cooking methods, and specific ingredients in each meal or snack.

**3.** Record any other factors that may impact digestion, such as stress levels, physical activity, or medication use.

## Experimenting with Elimination Diets:

**1.** Consider implementing an elimination diet under the guidance of a healthcare professional, such as a registered dietitian or nutritionist.

**2.**Start by eliminating common trigger foods such as dairy, gluten, soy, eggs, nuts, or certain additives and preservatives from your diet.

**3.**Gradually reintroduce eliminated foods one at a time while monitoring for any adverse reactions or symptoms.

**4.** Keep track of your body's responses to each reintroduced food to identify potential triggers for digestive discomfort.

## Seeking Guidance from Healthcare Professionals:

**1.** Consult with healthcare professionals, including dietitians and nutritionists, for personalised guidance and support in managing food intolerances and sensitivities.

**2.**Discuss your dietary history, symptoms, and goals with a healthcare provider to develop a tailored dietary strategy that addresses your individual needs.

**3.**Consider undergoing testing, such as food sensitivity testing or allergy testing, to identify specific triggers for your symptoms.

**4.** Work collaboratively with your healthcare team to implement dietary modifications and lifestyle changes that support optimal digestion and overall well-being.

By adopting proactive strategies for managing food intolerances and sensitivities, you can gain insight into your body's unique dietary needs and make informed choices that promote digestive health and comfort after gallbladder removal surgery. Remember to prioritise self-care, listen to your body's signals, and seek professional guidance when needed to optimise your postoperative dietary journey.

## Practical Tips for Dining Out and Social Settings After Gallbladder Removal

Dining out and attending social gatherings can present unique challenges for individuals adjusting to life after gallbladder removal surgery. However, with some practical tips and strategies, you can navigate these situations with confidence and ease:

**Navigating Restaurant Menus:**
**1.** Take time to review the restaurant menu in advance, if possible, to identify options that align with your dietary needs and preferences.
**2.** Look for dishes that are grilled, baked, steamed, or broiled, as these cooking methods typically involve less added fat.
**3.** Choose menu items that are rich in lean proteins, whole grains, and vegetables, while minimising heavy sauces, fried foods, and creamy dressings.

**Communicating Dietary Preferences and Restrictions:**
**1.** Don't hesitate to communicate your dietary preferences and restrictions to restaurant staff when ordering.
**2.** Ask questions about ingredients, cooking methods, and potential substitutions to ensure that your meal meets your needs.

**3.**Be polite but assertive in advocating for your dietary requirements, and don't feel pressured to order something that doesn't align with your health goals.

## Strategies for Enjoying Social Gatherings:

**1.**Plan ahead by eating a light snack or meal before attending social gatherings to curb hunger and prevent overindulgence.

**2.** Offer to bring a dish or snack that fits your dietary guidelines to share with others, ensuring that you have a safe and satisfying option available.

**3.** Focus on the social aspect of the gathering rather than solely on the food, and enjoy the company of friends and loved ones without feeling pressured to overeat.

## Being Proactive in Meal Planning:

**1.** Take a proactive approach to meal planning by preparing nutritious meals and snacks ahead of time.

**2.**Invest in portable containers and insulated bags to transport homemade meals and snacks when dining out or travelling.

**3.** Experiment with batch cooking and meal prepping to streamline the process of preparing healthy and convenient meals throughout the week.

By incorporating these practical tips into your dining-out experiences and social settings, you can enjoy delicious meals while adhering to your dietary guidelines and promoting digestive health after gallbladder removal surgery. Remember to be flexible, patient, and compassionate with yourself as you navigate these situations, and don't hesitate to seek support from friends, family members, or healthcare professionals when needed. With mindful choices and proactive planning, you can savor the pleasures of dining out and socialising while prioritising your health and well-being.

# CHAPTER THREE: TIPS FOR DIGESTIVE HEALTH AND COMFORT

Maintaining digestive health and comfort is a key focus as you navigate life after gallbladder removal surgery. In this chapter, we explore practical tips and strategies to support your digestive system, minimise discomfort, and foster overall well-being. From dietary considerations to lifestyle habits, these tips are designed to empower you with the knowledge needed to optimise your digestive health in the absence of a gallbladder.

## Mindful Eating Practices

Mindful eating is a powerful practice that can enhance your relationship with food, promote digestive health, and support overall well-being after gallbladder removal surgery. Here are some key principles to incorporate into your eating habits:
**Embracing Mindful Eating to Enhance Awareness:**

1.Cultivate mindfulness by tuning into your body's hunger and fullness cues before, during, and after meals.
2.Pause and check in with yourself before eating to assess your level of hunger and determine whether you're eating out of true physical hunger or other reasons, such as boredom or stress.

## Chewing Food Thoroughly for Digestive Health:

1.Take the time to chew your food thoroughly before swallowing. Chewing breaks down food into smaller particles, making it easier for your digestive system to process and absorb nutrients.
2. Aim to chew each bite of food at least 20-30 times to promote thorough digestion and optimise nutrient absorption.

## Avoiding Rushed or Distracted Eating:

1. Minimise distractions during meals by turning off electronic devices, avoiding work-related tasks, and focusing solely on the sensory experience of eating.

**2.**Eating slowly and mindfully allows you to savour the flavours, textures, and aromas of your food, leading to greater satisfaction and enjoyment.

**Taking Time to Savour and Enjoy Meals:**
**1.**Practise gratitude and appreciation for the nourishment that food provides to your body.
**2.**Engage your senses by noticing the colours, smells, tastes, and textures of the foods you're eating.
**3.**Foster a positive relationship with food by approaching meals with curiosity, openness, and non-judgment.

By incorporating mindful eating practices into your daily routine, you can develop a deeper connection to your body's needs, improve digestion, and prevent overeating and digestive discomfort. Remember that mindful eating is a skill that takes time and practice to cultivate, so be patient and compassionate with yourself as you explore this approach to nourishment and well-being. As you become more attuned to your body's signals and sensations, you'll find greater satisfaction and balance in your eating habits, supporting your journey toward optimal digestive health after gallbladder removal surgery.

## Balancing Macronutrients

Achieving a balance of macronutrients—proteins, carbohydrates, and fats—in your diet is essential for supporting overall health, promoting satiety, and optimizing digestion after gallbladder removal surgery. Here's how you can effectively balance macronutrients in your meals:

**Incorporating a Balanced Mix of Proteins, Carbohydrates, and Fats:**
1.Aim to include all three macronutrients—proteins, carbohydrates, and fats—in each meal to provide sustained energy and support various bodily functions.
2. Proteins are essential for muscle repair, immune function, and hormone

production, while carbohydrates serve as the body's primary source of energy. Healthy fats play a crucial role in supporting cell structure, hormone balance, and nutrient absorption.

**Choosing Lean Protein Sources, Whole Grains, and Healthy Fats:**
**1.** Select lean protein sources such as poultry, fish, tofu, tempeh, beans, and legumes to minimise saturated fat intake and promote muscle health.
**2.** Incorporate complex carbohydrates from whole grains like quinoa, brown rice, oats, barley, and whole wheat to provide fibre, vitamins, and minerals that support digestive health and satiety.
**3.** Choose healthy fats from sources such as avocados, nuts, seeds, olive oil, and fatty fish like salmon and mackerel to provide essential fatty acids and enhance flavour and texture in your meals.

**Monitoring Portion Sizes to Prevent Overconsumption:**
**1.** Be mindful of portion sizes to prevent overeating and reduce the risk of digestive

distress, particularly after gallbladder removal surgery.

2.Use visual cues such as your palm, fist, or thumb to estimate appropriate portion sizes for proteins, carbohydrates, and fats.

3.Practise mindful eating by paying attention to hunger and fullness cues, stopping when you feel satisfied rather than overly full.

By incorporating a balanced mix of proteins, carbohydrates, and fats into your meals and snacks, you can provide your body with the essential nutrients it needs to thrive while supporting optimal digestion and overall well-being. Experiment with different food combinations and portion sizes to find what works best for you, and remember to listen to your body's signals and adjust your dietary habits accordingly. With mindful choices and balanced nutrition, you can support your journey toward digestive health and vitality after gallbladder removal surgery.

# Managing Fibre Intake

Dietary fibre plays a crucial role in supporting digestive regularity, promoting satiety, and maintaining overall health after gallbladder removal surgery. Here are some key strategies for managing fibre intake effectively:

**Gradually Increasing Fibre Intake:**
**1.** Gradually increase your fibre intake over time to allow your digestive system to adapt. Start by incorporating small amounts of fibre-rich foods into your meals and gradually increase the quantity as tolerated.
**2.** Rapidly increasing fibre intake can lead to digestive discomfort, bloating, and gas, so it's essential to make dietary changes gradually and monitor your body's response.

**Including a Variety of Fiber-Rich Foods:**
**1.** Diversify your diet by including a variety of fibre-rich foods such as fruits, vegetables, whole grains, and legumes.

**2.** Choose fruits and vegetables with edible skins and seeds, as these parts are often rich in dietary fibre. Berries, apples, pears, broccoli, Brussels sprouts, carrots, and sweet potatoes are excellent choices.

**3.** Incorporate whole grains like quinoa, brown rice, oats, barley, and whole wheat into your meals to increase fibre intake and promote digestive health.

**4.** Experiment with legumes such as beans, lentils, chickpeas, and peas as plant-based sources of protein and fibre.

**Staying Hydrated:**

**1.** Drink plenty of water throughout the day to optimise the benefits of dietary fibre and prevent constipation.

**2.** Fibre absorbs water and adds bulk to stool, which helps promote regular bowel movements. However, inadequate hydration can lead to dry, hard stools and exacerbate digestive discomfort.

**3.** Aim to drink at least eight glasses of water daily, and consider increasing your fluid intake during periods of increased fiber consumption.

**Adjusting Fibre Intake Based on Individual Tolerance Levels:**

1.Pay attention to your body's response to dietary fibre and adjust your intake based on individual tolerance levels.

2.Some individuals may experience digestive discomfort or bloating when consuming certain types or amounts of fibre. If you experience discomfort, consider reducing your fibre intake temporarily and gradually reintroducing fibre-rich foods as tolerated.

3.Keep in mind that everyone's digestive system is unique, so it's essential to find a balance that works best for you.

By gradually increasing fibre intake, including a variety of fibre-rich foods in your diet, staying hydrated, and adjusting fibre intake based on individual tolerance levels, you can support optimal digestive health and well-being after gallbladder removal surgery. Be patient and mindful as you make dietary adjustments, and consult with healthcare professionals or registered dietitians for personalised guidance and support on your journey toward digestive wellness.

## Hydration Strategies

Maintaining adequate hydration is essential for supporting digestion, promoting overall health, and optimising recovery after gallbladder removal surgery. Here are some effective hydration strategies to incorporate into your daily routine:

**Drinking an Adequate Amount of Water Throughout the Day:**
**1.** Aim to drink enough water to stay hydrated throughout the day. The Institute of Medicine recommends approximately 9-13 cups (2.2-3 litres) of total fluids daily for most adults, but individual needs may vary based on factors such as age, gender, activity level, and climate.
**2.** Keep a water bottle with you throughout the day to remind yourself to drink regularly and stay hydrated.

**Limiting or Avoiding Caffeinated and Carbonated Beverages:**

1.Caffeinated and carbonated beverages, such as coffee, tea, soda, and energy drinks, can have diuretic effects and contribute to dehydration if consumed in excess.
2.Limit your intake of caffeinated and carbonated beverages, and consider choosing hydrating alternatives such as water, herbal teas, or diluted fruit juices.

**Consuming Clear Broths, Herbal Teas, and Water-Rich Foods:**
1.Incorporate clear broths, herbal teas, and water-rich fruits and vegetables into your diet to support hydration and add variety to your fluid intake.
2.Clear broths, such as chicken or vegetable broth, provide hydration along with electrolytes and minerals that support overall health.
3. Herbal teas, such as chamomile or peppermint tea, are caffeine-free options that can help hydrate the body and promote relaxation.
4.Water-rich fruits and vegetables, including cucumbers, watermelon, strawberries, oranges, and celery, are excellent sources of hydration and provide

additional vitamins, minerals, and antioxidants.

**Monitoring Urine Colour as a Hydration Indicator:**

**1.**Pay attention to the colour of your urine as a simple indicator of hydration status. Clear or light-coloured urine typically indicates adequate hydration, while dark-coloured urine may signal dehydration.

**2.**Aim for pale yellow urine as a general guideline, but keep in mind that certain medications, supplements, and foods can affect urine colour.

By incorporating these hydration strategies into your daily routine, you can support optimal digestion, promote overall health, and enhance recovery after gallbladder removal surgery. Remember to listen to your body's thirst cues, prioritise regular fluid intake, and make hydration a conscious part of your daily habits. If you have specific hydration needs or concerns, consult with healthcare professionals for personalised guidance and support on maintaining optimal hydration levels.

# Incorporating Digestive Aids

After gallbladder removal surgery, some individuals may experience digestive discomfort or irregularities as their bodies adjust to changes in bile production and digestion. Incorporating digestive aids into your routine can help soothe the digestive system, support nutrient absorption, and promote overall digestive health. Here are some effective digestive aids to consider:

**Exploring Natural Digestive Aids:**
**1.** Natural herbs and botanicals have long been used to alleviate digestive discomfort and promote gastrointestinal health. Ginger, peppermint, and chamomile are three examples of natural digestive aids that can help soothe digestive symptoms.
**2.**Ginger contains compounds that have been shown to stimulate digestive juices, improve digestion, and reduce nausea and inflammation in the digestive tract.
**3.** Peppermint has a calming effect on the muscles of the digestive system, which can

help relieve symptoms of indigestion, gas, bloating, and abdominal discomfort.

**4.** Chamomile is known for its anti-inflammatory and calming properties, making it beneficial for soothing gastrointestinal issues such as indigestion, cramping, and irritable bowel syndrome (IBS).

**Considering Digestive Enzyme Supplements:**

**1.**Digestive enzyme supplements can help support the breakdown of fats, proteins, and carbohydrates in the absence of a gallbladder, where bile storage and release are compromised.

**2.**Lipase, protease, and amylase are three common types of digestive enzymes that help break down fats, proteins, and carbohydrates, respectively.

**3.**Digestive enzyme supplements can be particularly beneficial for individuals who experience difficulty digesting fatty foods or who have symptoms of malabsorption after gallbladder removal surgery.

**Discussing the Use of Digestive Aids with Healthcare Professionals:**

**1.** Before incorporating digestive aids into your routine, it's essential to discuss your symptoms and concerns with healthcare professionals, such as your primary care physician, gastroenterologist, or registered dietitian.

**2.**Healthcare professionals can provide personalised recommendations based on your specific digestive issues, medical history, and nutritional needs.

**3.** They can also help you determine the appropriate dosage, timing, and duration of use for digestive aids and monitor your response to treatment over time.

Incorporating natural digestive aids such as ginger, peppermint, and chamomile into your diet, considering digestive enzyme supplements, and discussing the use of digestive aids with healthcare professionals can help alleviate digestive discomfort and promote optimal digestion and overall well-being after gallbladder removal surgery. Listen to your body's cues, be patient with the process of finding what works best for you, and work collaboratively with your healthcare team to address your digestive concerns effectively.

## Regular Physical Activity

Regular physical activity offers numerous benefits for digestive health, including improved bowel regularity, enhanced metabolism, and reduced risk of constipation and digestive discomfort. Aim for at least 30 minutes of moderate-intensity aerobic exercise most days of the week, as recommended by health guidelines. This can include activities such as brisk walking, cycling, swimming, or dancing.

In addition to aerobic exercise, incorporating strength training exercises two to three times per week can help build muscle mass, boost metabolism, and support overall physical function.

**Incorporating Gentle Activities to Enhance Digestion:**

**1.** Certain types of physical activity, such as walking, yoga, or gentle stretching exercises, can specifically target and support digestive health.

**2.** Walking after meals can help stimulate digestion, improve blood flow to the digestive organs, and prevent bloating and discomfort.

**3.**Yoga poses and stretches that focus on twisting and compressing the abdomen can help massage the internal organs, improve digestion, and alleviate symptoms of indigestion and gas.

## Being Mindful of Individual Energy Levels:

**1.** Listen to your body and be mindful of your individual energy levels when engaging in physical activity, especially during the recovery period after surgery.

**2.** Start gradually and progress slowly, gradually increasing the intensity and duration of your workouts as your strength and stamina improve.

**3.** Pay attention to how your body responds to different types of exercise and adjust the intensity and duration accordingly to prevent overexertion and fatigue.

Incorporating regular physical activity into your routine can not only support digestive health but also improve mood, reduce stress, and enhance overall quality of life. Choose activities that you enjoy and that fit into your lifestyle, and consider incorporating a variety of exercises to keep your routine interesting and engaging. Remember to stay hydrated, listen to your body's cues, and consult with healthcare professionals if you have any concerns or limitations regarding physical activity after gallbladder removal surgery. By making physical activity a priority, you can support your digestive health and well-being for the long term.

## Stress Management Techniques

Stress Management Techniques for Optimal Digestive Health After Gallbladder RemovalManaging stress is crucial for maintaining optimal digestive function and overall well-being, especially after gallbladder removal surgery. Here are some effective stress management techniques to consider:

**Prioritising Stress Management:**

**1.**Recognize the impact of stress on digestive health and prioritise stress management as an integral part of your overall wellness routine.

**2.**Chronic stress can exacerbate digestive symptoms such as indigestion, bloating, abdominal discomfort, and irregular bowel movements. By reducing stress levels, you can help alleviate these symptoms and support digestive well-being.

**Exploring Relaxation Techniques:**

**1.** Incorporate relaxation techniques into your daily routine to help reduce stress and promote relaxation. Deep breathing exercises, meditation, and progressive muscle relaxation are effective techniques for calming the mind and body.

**2.**Practise deep breathing by taking slow, deep breaths in through your nose, filling your lungs with air, and exhaling slowly through your mouth. Focus on the rhythm of your breath and let go of tension with each exhale.

**3.**Engage in mindfulness meditation practices that encourage present-moment awareness and non-judgmental acceptance of thoughts and sensations. Find a quiet, comfortable space to sit or lie down, and focus your attention on your breath or a specific point of focus.

**4.** Progressive muscle relaxation involves systematically tensing and relaxing different muscle groups in the body to release physical tension and promote relaxation. Start by tensing and then slowly releasing each muscle group, focusing on the sensations of relaxation as you let go of tension.

## Establishing a Consistent Sleep Routine:

**1.**Prioritise quality sleep as part of your stress management and digestive health regimen. Aim for 7-9 hours of restful sleep per night to support overall health and well-being.

**2.**Establish a consistent sleep routine by going to bed and waking up at the same time each day, even on weekends. Create a

relaxing bedtime routine that helps signal to your body that it's time to wind down.
**3.**Create a comfortable sleep environment by keeping your bedroom dark, cool, and quiet, and minimising exposure to screens and stimulating activities before bedtime.

By incorporating stress management techniques such as deep breathing, meditation, progressive muscle relaxation, and establishing a consistent sleep routine into your daily life, you can help reduce the impact of stress on digestive function and promote overall digestive health and well-being. Experiment with different techniques to find what works best for you, and make stress management a priority as you navigate the post-gallbladder removal recovery process. Remember that small, consistent efforts can make a significant difference in managing stress and supporting your digestive health in the long term.

# Gradual Introduction of Trigger Foods

Begin by reintroducing small amounts of potential trigger foods into your diet one at a time. This allows you to gauge your body's response and identify specific foods that may cause digestive discomfort.

Choose foods that you suspect may be triggers for symptoms such as bloating, gas, abdominal pain, diarrhoea, or nausea.

Common trigger foods after gallbladder removal include high-fat foods, spicy foods, caffeine, alcohol, and certain raw vegetables or fruits.

Start with a small portion of the trigger food and gradually increase the serving size over several days while monitoring your body's reactions.

**Monitoring Symptoms and Adjusting Your Diet:**

1.Keep a detailed record of your dietary intake and any associated symptoms in a food diary or journal. Note the type and amount of trigger food consumed, as well as

the timing and severity of any digestive
symptoms experienced.

**2.**Pay attention to subtle changes in your
body, including changes in bowel habits,
bloating, abdominal discomfort, or other
gastrointestinal symptoms.

**3.**If you experience digestive discomfort or
adverse reactions after consuming a
particular trigger food, consider reducing or
eliminating it from your diet and observe
how your symptoms evolve.

**Seeking Guidance from Healthcare
Professionals:**

**1.**If specific foods consistently cause
discomfort or exacerbate digestive
symptoms, consider seeking guidance from
healthcare professionals, such as a
gastroenterologist or registered dietitian.

**2.** Healthcare professionals can help you
identify potential trigger foods, develop
personalised dietary strategies, and explore
alternative options to meet your nutritional
needs.

**3.** They may recommend additional testing,
such as food sensitivity testing or allergy
testing, to pinpoint specific triggers for your

symptoms and guide your dietary modifications accordingly.

By gradually reintroducing trigger foods into your diet, monitoring symptoms, and seeking guidance from healthcare professionals as needed, you can gain valuable insights into your body's individual tolerance levels and make informed choices to support digestive wellness after gallbladder removal surgery. Remember to be patient and persistent in your approach, and prioritize self-care and mindful eating practices as you navigate the process of dietary adjustment and optimization.

By incorporating these tips for digestive health and comfort into your daily routine, you can promote a resilient and well-functioning digestive system. Remember that individual responses may vary, so it's essential to listen to your body, make adjustments as needed, and consult with healthcare professionals for personalised guidance on optimising your digestive well-being.

# CHAPTER FOUR: DELICIOUS RECIPES FOR GALLBLADDER-FRIENDL Y MEALS

Indulging in flavorful and nourishing meals is an essential aspect of maintaining a balanced diet and promoting digestive health after gallbladder removal surgery. In this chapter, we present a collection of delicious recipes tailored to support your dietary needs and preferences. From satisfying breakfast delights to hearty dinner creations, these recipes are designed to be gallbladder-friendly, easy to digest, and bursting with flavour.

## Breakfast Delights

**1. Banana Oat Pancakes**
**Ingredients:**
1 ripe banana, mashed
1/2 cup rolled oats
1 egg
1/4 teaspoon cinnamon
**Optional toppings: sliced strawberries, Greek yoghourt, honey**

Instructions:
1. In a bowl, combine mashed banana, rolled oats, egg, and cinnamon.
2. Heat a non-stick skillet over medium heat and lightly coat with cooking spray.
3. Pour pancake batter onto the skillet to form small pancakes.
4. Cook for 2-3 minutes on each side until golden brown and cooked through.
 5. Serve with your favourite toppings and enjoy!

## 2. Veggie Omelette

**Ingredients:**
2 eggs
Assorted vegetables (e.g., bell peppers, spinach, tomatoes)
1/4 cup shredded low-fat cheese
Salt and pepper to taste
Instructions:
1. In a bowl, beat the eggs until well combined. Season with salt and pepper.
2. Heat a non-stick skillet over medium heat and lightly coat with cooking spray.
3. Add the assorted vegetables to the skillet and sauté until tender.

4. Pour the beaten eggs over the vegetables and cook until the edges start to set.

5. Sprinkle shredded cheese over one half of the omelette and fold the other half over the filling.

6. Cook for an additional 1-2 minutes until the cheese melts.

7. Slide the omelette onto a plate, slice, and serve hot.

5.1. Breakfast Delights

Breakfast sets the tone for the day, providing essential nutrients and energy to fuel your activities. These breakfast delights are not only delicious but also gentle on your digestive system, making them ideal choices for those adjusting to life without a gallbladder.

**3.Egg Muffins with Vegetables**
**Ingredients:**
6 eggs
1/2 cup diced bell peppers
1/2 cup diced tomatoes
1/4 cup chopped spinach
Salt and pepper to taste
Instructions:

1. Preheat the oven to 350°F (175°C) and grease a muffin tin.
2. In a bowl, whisk together the eggs, salt, and pepper.
3. Stir in the diced bell peppers, tomatoes, and chopped spinach.
4. Pour the egg mixture evenly into the prepared muffin tin.
5. Bake for 20-25 minutes or until the egg muffins are set and lightly golden.
6. Allow to cool slightly before serving. These egg muffins can be stored in the refrigerator and reheated for a quick and nutritious breakfast throughout the week.

**4.Overnight Oats**
**Ingredients:**
1/2 cup rolled oats
1/2 cup almond milk (or any milk of your choice)
1 tablespoon chia seeds
1 tablespoon honey or maple syrup (optional)
1/4 cup mixed berries
Instructions:

1. In a jar or bowl, combine the rolled oats, almond milk, chia seeds, and honey or maple syrup if using.
2. Stir well to combine all ingredients.
3. Add the mixed berries on top of the oat mixture.
4. Cover and refrigerate overnight.
5. In the morning, give the oats a stir and enjoy cold or warm. Feel free to add additional toppings such as nuts, seeds, or a dollop of yoghourt for extra flavour and texture.

## 5.Smoothie Bowl

**Ingredients:**
1 frozen banana
1/2 cup frozen mixed berries
1/2 cup spinach or kale
1/2 cup almond milk (or any milk of your choice)
Toppings: sliced fresh fruits, granola, nuts, seeds, shredded coconut

**Instructions:**
1. In a blender, combine the frozen banana, frozen mixed berries, spinach or kale, and almond milk.
2. Blend until smooth and creamy.

3. Pour the smoothie into a bowl.
4. Arrange your favorite toppings on top of the smoothie bowl.
5. Serve immediately and enjoy this nutritious and refreshing breakfast option.

**6.Avocado Toast**

**Ingredients:**
1 ripe avocado
2 slices whole-grain bread, toasted
Salt and pepper to taste
Optional toppings: sliced tomatoes, microgreens, poached eggs
**Instructions:**
1. Mash the ripe avocado in a bowl until smooth.
2. Season with salt and pepper to taste.
3. Spread the mashed avocado evenly onto the toasted whole-grain bread slices.
4. Top with your favorite toppings such as sliced tomatoes, microgreens, or poached eggs.
5. Serve immediately and enjoy this simple yet satisfying breakfast option packed with healthy fats and fibre.

**7.Spinach and Feta Omelette**

**Ingredients:**
2 eggs
1/4 cup spinach leaves, chopped
2 tablespoons crumbled feta cheese
Salt and pepper to taste
1 teaspoon olive oil
**Instructions:**
1. In a bowl, whisk together eggs, chopped spinach, crumbled feta cheese, salt, and pepper.
2. Heat olive oil in a non-stick skillet over medium heat.
3. Pour the egg mixture into the skillet and cook until the edges begin to set.
4. Using a spatula, gently lift the edges of the omelette and tilt the skillet to allow the uncooked egg to flow to the bottom.
5. Once the omelette is set and the bottom is golden brown, fold it in half and slide onto a plate.
6. Serve hot with whole grain toast or a side of fresh fruit for a nutritious breakfast option.

## 8.Smoothie Bowl with Berries and Almond Butter.

**Ingredients:**

1 ripe banana, frozen
1/2 cup mixed berries (such as
strawberries, blueberries, raspberries)
1/2 cup spinach leaves
1/4 cup almond milk (or any milk of your
choice)
1 tablespoon almond butter
Toppings: sliced bananas, granola, chia
seeds, shredded coconut
**Instructions:**
1. In a blender, combine frozen banana,
mixed berries, spinach leaves, almond milk,
and almond butter.
2. Blend until smooth and creamy, adding
more almond milk if needed to reach
desired consistency.
3. Pour the smoothie into a bowl and top
with sliced bananas, granola, chia seeds,
and shredded coconut.
4. Enjoy with a spoon and savor the
delicious combination of flavors and
textures.

These breakfast delights are not only
nutritious and delicious but also gentle on
your digestive system, making them perfect
choices for starting your day off right after

gallbladder removal surgery. Feel free to customise these recipes according to your taste preferences and dietary needs, and enjoy the benefits of a wholesome breakfast to fuel your day ahead.

## Lunchtime Favourites

### 1. Quinoa Salad with Chickpeas and Vegetables

**Ingredients:**
1 cup cooked quinoa
1 can chickpeas, drained and rinsed
Assorted vegetables (e.g., cucumbers, cherry tomatoes, bell peppers)
Fresh herbs (e.g., parsley, mint, cilantro)
Lemon vinaigrette dressing

**Instructions:**
1. In a large bowl, combine cooked quinoa, chickpeas, chopped vegetables, and fresh herbs.
2. Drizzle with lemon vinaigrette dressing and toss to coat evenly.
3. Serve chilled or at room temperature as a refreshing and satisfying salad option.

### 2. Turkey and Avocado Wrap

**Ingredients:**

Whole-grain tortilla wraps
Sliced turkey breast
Sliced avocado
Lettuce leaves
Sliced tomatoes
Dijon mustard or hummus (optional)
**Instructions:**
1. Lay a whole-grain tortilla wrap flat on a clean surface.
2. Layer sliced turkey breast, avocado, lettuce leaves, and tomatoes on the tortilla.
3. Add a dollop of Dijon mustard or hummus for extra flavour (if desired).
4. Roll up the wrap tightly and slice in half diagonally.
5. Serve with a side of fresh fruit or vegetable sticks for a complete and satisfying meal.
Certainly! Here are some additional ideas for breakfast delights and lunchtime favourites:

### 3.Mediterranean Chickpea Salad
**Ingredients:**
1 can (15 ounces) chickpeas, drained and rinsed
1 cucumber, diced

1 cup cherry tomatoes, halved
1/4 cup red onion, finely chopped
1/4 cup Kalamata olives, pitted and sliced
2 tablespoons fresh parsley, chopped
Juice of 1 lemon
2 tablespoons extra virgin olive oil
 Salt and pepper to taste
 **Instructions:**
1. In a large bowl, combine chickpeas, diced cucumber, halved cherry tomatoes, chopped red onion, sliced Kalamata olives, and chopped parsley.
2. In a small bowl, whisk together lemon juice, extra virgin olive oil, salt, and pepper to make the dressing.
3. Pour the dressing over the salad ingredients and toss gently to coat evenly.
4. Chill in the refrigerator for at least 30 minutes to allow the flavors to meld.
5. Serve as a refreshing and nutritious lunch option, either on its own or alongside grilled chicken or fish.

**4.Caprese Quinoa Salad**
 **Ingredients:**
1 cup quinoa, cooked and cooled
1 cup cherry tomatoes, halved

1 cup fresh mozzarella balls (bocconcini),
halved
1/4 cup fresh basil leaves, torn
2 tablespoons extra virgin olive oil
1 tablespoon balsamic vinegar
 Salt and pepper to taste

**Instructions:**

1. In a large bowl, combine cooked quinoa, halved cherry tomatoes, halved mozzarella balls, and torn basil leaves.
2. In a small bowl, whisk together extra virgin olive oil, balsamic vinegar, salt, and pepper to make the dressing.
3. Drizzle the dressing over the quinoa salad and toss gently to combine.
4. Serve chilled or at room temperature as a light and flavorful lunch option, perfect for warm weather days.

## 5. Baked Salmon with Lemon and Herbs

**Ingredients:**
Salmon fillets
Fresh lemon slices
Fresh herbs (e.g., dill, parsley, thyme)
Olive oil
Salt and pepper to taste

**Instructions:**
1. Preheat the oven to 375°F (190°C) and line a baking sheet with parchment paper.
2. Place salmon fillets on the prepared baking sheet and season with salt and pepper.
3. Arrange lemon slices and fresh herbs on top of the salmon.
4. Drizzle with olive oil and bake for 12-15 minutes or until the salmon is cooked through and flakes easily with a fork.
5. Serve hot with steamed vegetables or a side salad for a nutritious and satisfying dinner option.

## 6.Vegetable Stir-Fry with Tofu
**Ingredients:**
Firm tofu, cubed
Assorted vegetables (e.g., broccoli, bell peppers, carrots, snap peas)
Garlic, minced
Low-sodium soy sauce or tamari
Sesame oil
Cooked brown rice or quinoa
**Instructions:**
1. Heat sesame oil in a large skillet or wok over medium heat.

2. Add cubed tofu to the skillet and cook until golden brown on all sides.
3. Add minced garlic and assorted vegetables to the skillet and stir-fry until tender-crisp.
4. Drizzle with low-sodium soy sauce or tamari and toss to coat evenly.
5. Serve vegetable stir-fry over cooked brown rice or quinoa for a satisfying and nutritious dinner option.

## Dinner Creations

Dinner is an opportunity to indulge in flavorful and nutritious meals that satisfy your appetite and nourish your body. These dinner creations are designed to be delicious, easy to prepare, and gentle on your digestive system, making them perfect options for post-gallbladder removal meals.

**1.Roasted Vegetable Quinoa Bowl**
  **Ingredients:**
1 cup quinoa, rinsed
 2 cups mixed vegetables (such as bell peppers, zucchini, carrots, cherry tomatoes)
2 tablespoons olive oil
2 cloves garlic, minced

1 teaspoon dried herbs (such as thyme, rosemary, or oregano)
Salt and pepper to taste
**Instructions:**
1. Preheat the oven to 400°F (200°C) and line a baking sheet with parchment paper.
2. In a bowl, toss the mixed vegetables with olive oil, minced garlic, dried herbs, salt, and pepper until evenly coated.
3. Spread the seasoned vegetables in a single layer on the prepared baking sheet.
4. Roast in the preheated oven for 20-25 minutes, or until the vegetables are tender and lightly browned.
5. While the vegetables are roasting, cook the quinoa according to package instructions.
6. Serve the roasted vegetables over a bed of cooked quinoa for a hearty and nutritious dinner option.

## 2.Herb-Crusted Baked Chicken

**Ingredients**
2 boneless, skinless chicken breasts
1/4 cup breadcrumbs (preferably whole wheat)
2 tablespoons grated Parmesan cheese

1 teaspoon dried Italian herbs (such as basil, oregano, thyme)
1 tablespoon olive oil
 Salt and pepper to taste

**Instructions:**

1. Preheat the oven to 375°F (190°C) and line a baking dish with parchment paper.
2. In a shallow bowl, combine breadcrumbs, grated Parmesan cheese, dried herbs, salt, and pepper.
3. Brush each chicken breast with olive oil, then dredge in the breadcrumb mixture, pressing gently to adhere.
4. Place the coated chicken breasts in the prepared baking dish.
5. Bake in the preheated oven for 25-30 minutes, or until the chicken is cooked through and golden brown.
6. Serve the herb-crusted baked chicken with steamed vegetables or a side salad for a satisfying and protein-rich dinner.

These dinner creations offer a balance of flavours and nutrients while being gentle on your digestive system. Experiment with different ingredients and flavour combinations to keep your meals exciting and enjoyable. Remember to listen to your body and make adjustments as needed to suit your individual preferences and dietary requirements.

## Snacks and Sides

### 1. Greek Yoghourt Parfait

**Ingredients:**
Plain Greek yoghourt
 Fresh berries (e.g., strawberries, blueberries, raspberries)
Granola or toasted oats
 Honey or maple syrup (optional)
 **Instructions:**
1. Layer plain Greek yoghourt, fresh berries, and granola in a glass or bowl.
2. Drizzle with honey or maple syrup for added sweetness (if desired).
3. Enjoy as a nutritious and satisfying snack or light dessert option.

### 2.Avocado Toast with Cherry Tomatoes

**Ingredients:**
2 slices whole grain bread, toasted
1 ripe avocado, mashed
1/2 cup cherry tomatoes, halved

Sprinkle of sea salt and black pepper
Optional: drizzle of balsamic glaze or olive oil

**Instructions:**

1. Spread mashed avocado evenly onto the toasted whole grain bread slices.
2. Top with halved cherry tomatoes, and season with a sprinkle of sea salt and black pepper.
3. For added flavour, drizzle with balsamic glaze or olive oil if desired.
4. Serve as a nutritious and satisfying snack or side dish.

## 3.Vegetable Crudité with Hummus

**Ingredients:**

Assorted raw vegetables (such as carrot sticks, cucumber slices, bell pepper strips, cherry tomatoes, celery sticks)
Homemade or store-bought hummus

**Instructions:**

1. Wash and prepare the raw vegetables by cutting them into bite-sized sticks or slices.
2. Arrange the vegetable crudité on a platter or serving dish.
3. Serve with a side of hummus for dipping.

4. Enjoy this crunchy and nutrient-rich snack or side option.

**4.Quinoa and Black Bean Salad**
**Ingredients:**
1 cup cooked quinoa, cooled
1 can (15 ounces) black beans, drained and rinsed
1/2 cup diced red bell pepper
1/2 cup diced cucumber
1/4 cup chopped fresh cilantro
Juice of 1 lime
2 tablespoons olive oil
Salt and pepper to taste
**Instructions:**
1. In a large bowl, combine cooked quinoa, black beans, diced red bell pepper, diced cucumber, and chopped fresh cilantro.
2. In a small bowl, whisk together lime juice, olive oil, salt, and pepper to create the dressing.
3. Pour the dressing over the quinoa and black bean mixture, and toss to coat evenly.
4. Chill in the refrigerator for at least 30 minutes before serving.
5. Serve as a refreshing and protein-packed side dish or snack option.

**5.Baked Sweet Potato Fries**
**Ingredients:**
2 medium sweet potatoes, peeled and cut
into fries
1 tablespoon olive oil
1 teaspoon paprika
1/2 teaspoon garlic powder
1/2 teaspoon sea salt
Freshly ground black pepper to taste
**Instructions**
1. Preheat the oven to 425°F (220°C) and
line a baking sheet with parchment paper.
2. In a large bowl, toss the sweet potato
fries with olive oil, paprika, garlic powder,
sea salt, and black pepper until evenly
coated.
3. Spread the seasoned sweet potato fries in
a single layer on the prepared baking sheet.
4. Bake in the preheated oven for 20-25
minutes, flipping halfway through, until the
fries are golden brown and crispy.
5. Serve hot as a wholesome and flavorful
snack or side dish.

These snacks and sides offer a variety of
flavours, textures, and nutrients to
complement your meals and keep you

satisfied throughout the day. Feel free to customise the recipes according to your taste preferences and dietary needs. Enjoy exploring new flavour combinations and incorporating wholesome ingredients into your snacks and side dishes.

# CHAPTER FIVE: COPING WITH CHALLENGES AND COMMON CONCERNS

Navigating life after gallbladder removal surgery may present various challenges and common concerns as you adjust to dietary modifications, manage potential digestive issues, and adapt to lifestyle changes. This chapter explores practical strategies and coping mechanisms to address these challenges effectively, promote resilience, and enhance overall well-being in your postoperative journey.

## Managing Digestive Discomfort

Managing digestive discomfort effectively involves recognizing common symptoms, implementing dietary modifications, and adopting mindful eating practices to support digestion. Here's a deeper dive into managing digestive discomfort:

**Recognizing Common Digestive Symptoms:**

1. Common digestive symptoms after gallbladder removal surgery include bloating, gas, diarrhoea, indigestion, and abdominal discomfort.

2.Understanding the potential triggers for these symptoms, such as high-fat foods, spicy foods, caffeine, alcohol, and certain raw vegetables or fruits, can help you identify patterns and make informed dietary choices.

**Implementing Dietary Modifications:**

1. Reduce fat intake by choosing lean protein sources, such as poultry, fish, tofu, and legumes, and opting for cooking methods like baking, grilling, or steaming instead of frying.

2.Avoid spicy foods, acidic foods, and carbonated beverages, which can irritate the digestive tract and exacerbate symptoms.

3.Incorporate digestive-friendly foods such as cooked vegetables, fruits without skins, whole grains, and low-fat dairy products to promote digestion and minimize discomfort.

4. Experiment with lactose-free or gluten-free alternatives if you suspect lactose or gluten intolerance is contributing to your symptoms.

## Experimenting with Small, Frequent Meals:

1. Consuming small, frequent meals throughout the day rather than large, heavy meals can help prevent overloading the digestive system and minimise symptoms.
2.Space meals evenly throughout the day and include a balance of protein, carbohydrates, and fibre-rich foods to promote satiety and support digestion.
3. Practise mindful eating by chewing food thoroughly, eating slowly, and paying attention to hunger and fullness cues. Avoid rushing through meals or eating while distracted, as this can hinder proper digestion and exacerbate symptoms.

## Incorporating Stress Management Techniques:

1.Stress can exacerbate digestive symptoms, so incorporating stress management techniques such as deep

breathing, meditation, and gentle exercise
can help alleviate discomfort.
2.Prioritise adequate sleep, engage in
regular physical activity, and make time for
relaxation activities to support overall
well-being and digestive health.

**Seeking Professional Guidance:**
1.If digestive symptoms persist or worsen
despite dietary modifications and lifestyle
changes, consider seeking guidance from
healthcare professionals such as a
gastroenterologist or registered dietitian.
2.Healthcare professionals can help identify
underlying causes of digestive discomfort,
recommend appropriate diagnostic tests,
and develop personalised treatment plans
tailored to your individual needs.

# Addressing Dietary Adjustments After Gallbladder Removal Surgery

After gallbladder removal surgery, adopting
dietary adjustments is essential for
supporting digestive health and overall

well-being. Here's how to address dietary adjustments effectively:

**Embracing Dietary Changes:**
1.Embrace dietary changes that focus on reducing fat intake, increasing fibre consumption, and moderating portion sizes to support digestive function and minimise discomfort.
2.Incorporate lean protein sources such as poultry, fish, tofu, and legumes, and opt for cooking methods like baking, grilling, or steaming instead of frying.
3. Increase fibre consumption by incorporating fruits, vegetables, whole grains, and legumes into your meals to promote regular bowel movements and support digestive health.

**Seeking Guidance from Healthcare Professionals:**
1.Seek guidance from healthcare professionals, dietitians, or nutritionists to develop personalised meal plans and dietary strategies tailored to your individual needs, preferences, and health goals.

2.Healthcare professionals can provide valuable insight into managing dietary adjustments after gallbladder removal surgery, including recommendations for specific foods to include or avoid, portion control strategies, and meal timing considerations.

**Exploring Alternative Cooking Methods and Ingredient Substitutions:**

1.Explore alternative cooking methods such as baking, grilling, steaming, or sautéing with minimal oil to reduce fat content in meals while retaining flavour and moisture.

2. Experiment with ingredient substitutions to replace high-fat or potentially irritating foods with healthier alternatives. For example, use Greek yoghourt instead of sour cream, applesauce instead of oil in baking, or herbs and spices for flavour instead of salt.

3. Incorporate flavour-enhancing techniques such as marinating meats, using citrus juices or vinegar-based dressings, and adding fresh herbs and spices to

enhance the taste of dishes without relying on excessive fats or salt.

**Maintaining Enjoyment and Satisfaction with Meals:**
1.Focus on creating balanced meals that are both nutritious and delicious, incorporating a variety of colours, textures, and flavours to keep meals interesting and satisfying.
2.Be open to trying new foods, recipes, and culinary techniques to maintain enjoyment and satisfaction with your meals while adhering to dietary adjustments.
3. Involve family members or friends in meal planning and preparation to foster a supportive and enjoyable dining experience.

By embracing dietary changes, seeking guidance from healthcare professionals, exploring alternative cooking methods and ingredient substitutions, and maintaining enjoyment and satisfaction with meals, you can effectively address dietary adjustments after gallbladder removal surgery and support digestive health and overall well-being in the long term. Remember to listen to your body's cues, be patient with the adjustment process, and celebrate progress and successes along the way.

## Coping with Emotional and Psychological Effects After Gallbladder Removal Surgery

The emotional and psychological effects of gallbladder removal surgery can be significant, as individuals navigate changes to their bodies and lifestyles. Here are some strategies to help cope with these effects effectively:

**Acknowledging and Validating Emotional Responses:**
1.It's essential to acknowledge and validate the range of emotions that may arise after gallbladder removal surgery, including anxiety, frustration, sadness, or uncertainty about the future.
2. Understand that it's normal to experience a variety of emotions during the recovery process, and allow yourself the time and space to process these feelings without judgement.

**Engaging in Self-Care Practices:**
1.Incorporate self-care practices into your daily routine to manage stress and promote emotional well-being. Mindfulness meditation, deep breathing exercises, progressive muscle relaxation, or journaling can help calm the mind, reduce anxiety, and foster a sense of inner peace.
2.Make time for activities that bring you joy and relaxation, whether it's spending time in nature, listening to music, practising hobbies, or indulging in creative outlets.

**Seeking Support from Others:**
1.Reach out to friends, family members, or support groups for individuals who have undergone similar experiences to share stories, offer encouragement, and provide reassurance.
2. Connecting with others who can empathise with your situation can help reduce feelings of isolation and loneliness and provide a sense of camaraderie and understanding.
3.Consider joining online forums, support groups, or community organisations

dedicated to supporting individuals undergoing surgery or managing chronic health conditions.

## Communicating with Healthcare Providers:

1.Don't hesitate to communicate openly and honestly with your healthcare providers about any emotional or psychological challenges you may be facing.
2. Your healthcare team can offer support, guidance, and resources to help you cope with emotional distress and address any concerns or questions you may have about your recovery process.

## Maintaining a Positive Outlook:

1. Focus on maintaining a positive outlook and celebrating small victories and milestones along the way.
2.Practise gratitude for the progress you've made and the support you've received from loved ones and healthcare professionals throughout your recovery journey.

Remember that healing takes time, both physically and emotionally, and it's okay to seek help and support when needed. By acknowledging your emotional responses, engaging in self-care practices, seeking support from others, communicating with healthcare providers, and maintaining a positive outlook, you can navigate the emotional and psychological effects of gallbladder removal surgery with resilience and grace. Allow yourself the grace to heal at your own pace and trust that brighter days lie ahead.

## Adapting to Lifestyle Changes After Gallbladder Removal Surgery

Navigating life after gallbladder removal surgery often involves adapting to various lifestyle changes. Here's how you can effectively adjust to these changes and promote your overall health and well-being:

**Embracing Lifestyle Adjustments:**
1. Embrace lifestyle adjustments that prioritise your health and well-being, such as incorporating regular physical activity,

maintaining adequate hydration, and
practising stress management techniques.
2.Aim for at least 30 minutes of
moderate-intensity exercise most days of
the week, whether it's walking, swimming,
yoga, or cycling. Physical activity not only
supports digestive health but also improves
mood, boosts energy levels, and enhances
overall fitness.
3. Stay hydrated by drinking plenty of water
throughout the day, as adequate hydration
is essential for digestion, metabolism, and
overall cellular function.
4. Practice stress management techniques
such as deep breathing, meditation,
mindfulness, or progressive muscle
relaxation to reduce stress levels and
promote relaxation.

**Exploring Relaxation Techniques and
Hobbies:**
1. Explore relaxation techniques and
hobbies that bring joy, fulfilment, and a
sense of balance to your life. Engage in
activities such as gardening, painting,
listening to music, reading, or spending
time in nature.

2. Find activities that resonate with you and allow you to unwind, recharge, and reconnect with yourself. Cultivate hobbies that provide a sense of purpose and contribute to your overall well-being.

**Prioritising Self-Care Practices:**
1.Prioritise self-care practices that nourish your body, mind, and spirit. Set aside time each day for activities that promote relaxation, self-reflection, and personal growth.
2. Practise self-compassion and kindness towards yourself as you navigate the recovery process. Be patient with yourself and allow yourself the grace to adapt to changes at your own pace.
3. Set realistic expectations for recovery and adjustment to postoperative life. Recognize that healing takes time, and it's normal to experience ups and downs along the way.

**Seeking Support and Connection:**
1.Seek support and connection from friends, family members, support groups, or online communities who can offer

encouragement, understanding, and
empathy.
2.Share your experiences, challenges, and
triumphs with others who have undergone
similar journeys. Connecting with others
who can relate to your experiences can
provide validation, reassurance, and a
sense of belonging.

By embracing lifestyle adjustments,
exploring relaxation techniques and
hobbies, prioritising self-care practices, and
seeking support and connection, you can
adapt to life after gallbladder removal
surgery with resilience and grace.
Remember to listen to your body's needs,
honor your emotions, and celebrate the
progress you've made along the way. With
time, patience, and self-care, you can
cultivate a fulfilling and vibrant life that
supports your overall health and
well-being.

# Fostering Resilience and Optimism After Gallbladder Removal Surgery

Recovering from gallbladder removal surgery can present numerous challenges, but fostering resilience and optimism can empower you to navigate the journey with grace and determination. Here's how you can cultivate resilience and optimism:

**Cultivating Resilience:**
1.Cultivate resilience by recognizing and drawing upon your strengths, coping mechanisms, and adaptive strategies to overcome challenges and setbacks. Reflect on past experiences where you've demonstrated resilience and use those as sources of inspiration and guidance.
2.Embrace the belief that challenges are opportunities for growth and learning. Approach setbacks with a mindset of curiosity and openness to new possibilities.
3. Build a support network of friends, family members, and healthcare professionals who can offer encouragement, guidance, and practical

assistance as you navigate the recovery process.

**Practising Gratitude, Mindfulness, and Self-Compassion:**

1.Practise gratitude by focusing on the positive aspects of your life and expressing appreciation for the blessings, big and small, that surround you. Cultivating a sense of gratitude can shift your perspective and foster a greater sense of well-being.

2. Embrace mindfulness by staying present in the moment and cultivating awareness of your thoughts, feelings, and sensations without judgement. Mindfulness practices such as meditation, deep breathing, or body scans can help reduce stress, enhance self-awareness, and promote emotional resilience.

3.Practise self-compassion by treating yourself with kindness, understanding, and acceptance, especially during times of difficulty or challenge. Recognize that you are doing the best you can with the resources and circumstances available to you.

**Celebrating Progress and Small Victories:**

1. Celebrate progress, small victories, and moments of resilience as you navigate the journey of recovery and adjustment after gallbladder removal surgery. Recognize and acknowledge your accomplishments, no matter how small they may seem.

2.Keep a journal or gratitude log to document moments of resilience, progress, and gratitude. Reflecting on your experiences can help reinforce a positive outlook and provide motivation during challenging times.

3. Surround yourself with positivity and inspiration. Seek out stories of resilience and triumph, engage in activities that uplift and energise you, and cultivate an environment that fosters optimism and hope.

By cultivating resilience, practising gratitude, mindfulness, and self-compassion, and celebrating progress and small victories, you can foster a positive outlook and sense of empowerment as you navigate the journey of recovery and adjustment after gallbladder removal surgery. Remember that resilience is a skill that can be developed and strengthened over time, and with patience, perseverance, and self-care, you can emerge from adversity stronger, wiser, and more resilient than ever before.

By implementing these coping strategies and seeking support from healthcare professionals and support networks, you can effectively manage challenges, address common concerns, and cultivate resilience in your postoperative journey. Remember that it's normal to experience ups and downs along the way, and prioritising self-care and self-compassion can help you navigate the path toward optimal health and well-being after gallbladder surgery.

# CONCLUSION: EMBRACING A VIBRANT LIFESTYLE WITHOUT A GALLBLADDER

Embarking on the journey of life without a gallbladder may initially pose challenges, but it is a path paved with opportunities for newfound wellness, resilience, and vitality. Throughout this guide, we have explored the intricacies of post-gallbladder removal living, offering insights, strategies, and practical tips to support your physical and emotional well-being.

The absence of a gallbladder calls for adjustments, particularly in dietary habits and lifestyle choices. From understanding the surgical process to embracing a balanced diet and navigating potential challenges, you have acquired the knowledge needed to make informed decisions about your health. It's crucial to remember that each individual's experience is unique, and the key to a vibrant lifestyle lies in your ability to adapt, listen to your body, and cultivate a sense of empowerment over your well-being.

Meal planning strategies, coping mechanisms for common concerns, and the importance of professional guidance have been highlighted to provide you with a comprehensive toolkit for success. By incorporating these insights into your daily life, you can not only manage the specific challenges associated with gallbladder removal but also embark on a journey toward optimal health and a vibrant, fulfilling lifestyle.

As you move forward, keep in mind the significance of self-compassion, resilience, and the celebration of small victories. Embrace the support of healthcare professionals, connect with communities that share similar experiences, and honor the uniqueness of your own path. The road to vibrant living after gallbladder surgery is a journey that invites continuous learning, adaptation, and a commitment to prioritising your health.

In closing, the absence of a gallbladder does not define your wellness; rather, it opens the door to a lifestyle characterised by balance, mindfulness, and a renewed appreciation for the resilience of the human body. With informed choices, a positive mindset, and a commitment to self-care, you can embrace a vibrant, fulfilling life without a gallbladder—a life that thrives in the face of change and radiates with the energy of well-being.